I0693445

INTRODUCTION ON SAXENDA

Saxenda is an injectable prescription remedy particularly authorised for weight control alongside dietary adjustments and accelerated bodily hobby for certain adults with extra weight. Saxenda carries liraglutide, a drug classified as a glucagon-like peptide (GLP-1) agonist. Saxenda is a persistent weight management medicine. "Like different continual sicknesses, weight problems treatment wishes to be lifelong," says Elizabeth Mann, M.D., a pediatric endocrinologist at UW Health Kids in Wisconsin. She explains that Saxenda doesn't fundamentally alternate the underlying causes of obesity—it best facilitates control it. Additionally, Saxenda is not a substitute for weight reduction surgical operation, says Seth Kipnis, M.D., the medical director of bariatric and robot surgical operation at Jersey Shore University Medical Center. "It can supplement [surgery] or be used for patients who aren't eligible for weight-loss surgical operation," he adds.

HOW DOES SAXENDA WORK?

Chemically, GLP-1 agonists like Saxenda are designed to mimic the consequences of GLP-1—a hormone your frame releases after you consume. Saxenda acts like GLP-1 by triggering a satiety signal to your brain and slowing down motion on your gut. The net effect is feeling extra full and much less hungry. The herbal shape of GLP-1, but, most effective remains on your device for a few minutes. Saxenda is damaged down more slowly, making an allowance for a sustained effect over the path of an afternoon.

percentile or extra for age and intercourse, says Dr. Mann. The producer labeling additionally includes a minimal pediatric weight requirement above 132 kilos. Saxenda is not encouraged for individuals with a non-public or own family history of medullary thyroid most cancers, says Dr. Mann, and in human beings with a rare, hereditary endocrine sickness called multiple endocrine neoplasia (MEN 2). "It is also contraindicated in being pregnant," she says. According to the manufacturer (Novo Nordisk), Saxenda additionally hasn't been studied for use in the course of lactation. Always consult your health practitioner approximately any issues you can have earlier than beginning a brand new remedy.

- Liver disorder

- Previous swelling of the tongue, face, or lips with difficulty respiration, issue swallowing, hoarseness, or tightening of the throat

- Stomach troubles

- Suicidal thoughts, plans, or try; a preceding suicide try with the aid of you or a family member

- Thyroid cancer or if a person on your family had thyroid most cancers

- An uncommon or hypersensitive reaction to

liraglutide, other medicinal drugs, foods, dyes, or preservatives

•	Pregnant or looking to get pregnant

•	Breast-feeding

HOW OUGHT TO I USE THIS MEDICINE?

This remedy is for injection below the pores and skin of your top leg, belly place, or top arm. You might be taught how to prepare and deliver this medication. Use precisely as directed. Take your medicinal drug at everyday durations. Do no longer take it extra regularly than directed. This remedy comes with INSTRUCTIONS FOR USE. Ask your pharmacist for instructions on a way to use this medicinal drug. Read the data cautiously. Talk to your pharmacist or care group when you have questions.

It is vital that you placed your used needles and syringes in a unique sharps field. Do no longer position them in a trash can. If you do not have a sharps container, call your pharmacist or care crew to get one. A unique MedGuide may be given to you by using the pharmacist with every prescription and replenish. Be certain to examine these records cautiously on every occasion. Talk in your care crew about the use of this medicine in kids. While it can be prescribed for kids as younger as 12 years of age for selected conditions, precautions do apply.

Overdosage: If you think you have got taken too much of this medicine touch a poison control center or emergency room without delay. NOTE: This remedy is handiest for you. Do now not proportion this medicine with others.

WHAT MUST I WATCH FOR AT THE SAME TIME AS USING THIS MEDICINE?

Visit your care team for normal assessments on your progress. Drink plenty of fluids at the same time as taking this medicinal drug. Check along with your care team in case you get an assault of intense diarrhea, nausea, and vomiting. The loss of an excessive amount of body fluid could make it dangerous for you to take this remedy. This medicinal drug may affect blood sugar ranges. Ask your care crew if changes in food regimen or medications are wanted when you have diabetes.

Patients and their households must watch out for worsening depression or mind of suicide. Also watch out for surprising changes in feelings including feeling worrying, agitated, panicky, irritable, antagonistic, competitive, impulsive, critically stressed, overly excited and hyperactive, or no longer being able to sleep. If this occurs, mainly at the beginning of treatment or after an alternate in dose, call your care group. Women must tell their care team in the event that they wish to grow to be pregnant or assume they might be pregnant. Losing weight whilst pregnant isn't always recommended and may reason damage to the unborn infant. Talk on your care team for greater facts.

WHAT FACET CONSEQUENCES MAY ALSO I NOTE FROM RECEIVING THIS MEDICATION?

Side consequences which you have to document on your care group as quickly as possible:

- Allergic reactions or angioedema—pores and skin rash, itching, and hives, swelling of the face, eyes, lips, tongue, fingers, or legs, problem swallowing or breathing

- Fast or abnormal heartbeat

- Gallbladder issues—excessive stomach pain, nausea, vomiting, fever

- Kidney damage—decrease in the quantity of urine, swelling of the ankles, palms, or ft

- Pancreatitis—intense stomach ache that spreads for your lower back or receives worse after ingesting or whilst touched, fever, nausea, vomiting

- Thoughts of suicide or self-harm, worsening temper, emotions of melancholy

- Thyroid most cancers—new mass or lump in the neck, ache or trouble swallowing, trouble respiration, hoarseness

Side consequences that usually do not require scientific attention (report to your care crew if they retain or are bothersome):

- Constipation

- Dizziness

- Fatigue

- Headache

- Loss of Appetite

- Nausea

- Upset belly

This listing might not describe all feasible aspect outcomes. Call your physician for scientific advice approximately aspect consequences. You may additionally report facet consequences to FDA at 1-800-FDA-1088.

WHERE SHOULD I KEEP MY MEDICINE?

Keep out of the reach of kids and pets. Store unopened pen in a refrigerator among 2 and 8 tiers C (36 and forty six degrees F). Do now not freeze or use if the medication has been frozen. Protect from light and immoderate warmness. After you first use the pen, it could be saved at room temperature among 15 and 30 stages C (fifty nine and 86 degrees F) or in a fridge. Throw away your used pen after 30 days or after the expiration date, whichever comes first.

Do no longer keep your pen with the needle attached. If the needle is left on, medicine might also leak from the pen. NOTE: This sheet is a precis. It might not cover all feasible facts. If you've got questions about this medicine, communicate to your doctor, pharmacist, or health care issuer.

WHAT MAY ADDITIONALLY ENGAGE WITH THIS REMEDY?

• Insulin and different medications for diabetes

This listing may not describe all possible interactions. Give your health care issuer a list of all the drugs, herbs, non-pharmaceuticals, or dietary dietary supplements you use. Also inform them in case you smoke, drink alcohol, or use illegal pills. Some objects may also engage with your medicinal drug.

HOW NEED TO I USE SAXENDA?

Saxenda is commonly given as soon as in step with day. Follow all guidelines in your prescription label. Your doctor may also once in a while alternate your dose. Do not use this remedy in larger or smaller quantities or for longer than endorsed. Do not use Saxenda and Victoza together. These brands incorporate the same energetic component however they need to no longer be used collectively. Read all affected person records, medicinal drug courses, and coaching sheets furnished to you. Ask your doctor or pharmacist if you have any questions. Saxenda is injected beneath the pores and skin at any time of the day, with or without a meal. You can be proven the way to use injections at domestic. Do now not self-inject this medicine in case you do not recognize how to supply the injection and nicely take away used needles and syringes. Saxenda is available in a prefilled injection pen. Ask your pharmacist which sort of needles is great to use along with your pen. Your care provider will display you the nice places in your frame to inject Saxenda. Use a unique location on every occasion you supply an injection. Do not inject into the same region instances in a row. Do not use Saxenda if it has modified colors or if it has particles in it. Call your pharmacist for brand spanking new medicine. Also watch for signs of high blood sugar (hyperglycemia) which include elevated thirst or urination, blurred imaginative and prescient, headache, and tiredness. Blood sugar degrees can be affected by stress, illness, surgery, exercising, alcohol use, or skipping meals. Ask your health practitioner before changing your dose or medicinal drug agenda.

Use a disposable needle simplest once. Follow any nation or nearby legal guidelines approximately throwing away used needles and syringes. Use a puncture-proof "sharps" disposal box (ask your pharmacist wherein to get one and the way to throw it away). Keep this box out of the attain of children and pets. Saxenda is only a part of a complete remedy program which can additionally encompass weight loss program, exercising, weight manage, normal blood sugar checking out, and unique hospital therapy. Follow your medical doctor's instructions very closely.

Storing unopened injection pens: Store within the refrigerator. Do now not freeze Saxenda, and throw away the medicine if it has become frozen. Do not use an unopened injection pen if the expiration date at the label has exceeded. Storing after your first use: You may additionally keep "in-use" injection pens inside the refrigerator or at room temperature. Protect the pens from moisture, warmness, and sunlight. Use within 30 days. Remove the needle earlier than storing an injection pen, and keep the cap at the pen when not in use.

SAXENDA SIDE OUTCOMES

Get emergency scientific help when you have signs and symptoms of an allergic reaction to Saxenda: hives; fast heartbeats; dizziness; trouble breathing or swallowing; swelling of your face, lips, tongue, or throat. Call your health practitioner straight away if you have:

- racing or pounding heartbeats;

- Sudden changes in temper or conduct, suicidal mind;

- Excessive ongoing nausea, vomiting, or diarrhea;

- Symptoms of a thyroid tumor - swelling or a lump in your neck, problem swallowing, a hoarse voice, feeling quick of breathe;

- Gallbladder troubles - fever, upper belly pain, clay-coloured stools, jaundice (yellowing of your pores and skin or eyes);

- symptoms of pancreatitis - intense ache on your higher belly spreading for your again, nausea without or with vomiting, speedy coronary heart rate;

- critically low blood sugar - excessive weak spot, confusion, tremors, sweating, fast heart fee, problem talking, nausea, vomiting, rapid breathing, fainting, and seizure (convulsions); or

•	Kidney troubles - very little urination; painful or difficult urination; swelling in your feet or ankles; feeling tired or quick of breath.

Common Saxenda side consequences may additionally consist of:

•	Nausea (especially when you start the use of Saxenda), vomiting, belly pain;

•	extended coronary heart rate;

- Diarrhea, constipation;

- Headache, dizziness; or

- Feeling tired.

This is not a whole listing of facet consequences and others can also arise. Call your doctor for clinical advice about aspect results. You may also record aspect consequences to FDA at 1-800-FDA-1088.

WHAT DIFFERENT TABLETS WILL HAVE AN EFFECT ON SAXENDA?

Saxenda can slow your digestion, and it can take longer on your frame to absorb any drugs you are taking by way of mouth.

Tell your medical doctor about all of your current medicines and any you begin or stop the use of, specifically:

- Insulin; or

- Oral diabetes remedy - Glucotrol, Metaglip, Amaryl, Avandaryl, Duetact, DiaBeta, Micronase, Glucovance, and others.

This list isn't always complete. Other tablets may additionally interact with liraglutide, such as prescription and over-the-counter drugs, vitamins, and herbal products. Not all possible interactions are listed in this medicine manual.

WARNINGS

The Victoza logo of liraglutide is used collectively with diet and exercising to deal with kind 2 diabetes. Do now not use Saxenda and Victoza collectively. You should not use Saxenda when you have more than one endocrine neoplasia type 2 (tumors for your glands), a personal or family records of medullary thyroid most cancers, insulin-dependent diabetes, diabetic ketoacidosis, or are pregnant. In animal studies, liraglutide prompted thyroid tumors or thyroid most cancers. It isn't recognised whether or not these outcomes might arise in people using regular doses. Call your physician right away if you have signs of a thyroid tumor, along with swelling or a lump in your neck, hassle swallowing, a hoarse voice, or shortness of breath.

BEFORE USING SAXENDA

You have to no longer use Saxenda if you are allergic to liraglutide, or if you have:

•	Multiple endocrine neoplasia type 2 (tumors in your glands);

•	a private or circle of relatives records of medullary thyroid carcinoma (a form of thyroid cancer); or

•	Diabetic ketoacidosis (name your health practitioner for remedy).

You should now not use Saxenda if you also use insulin or other drugs like liraglutide (albiglutide, dulaglutide, exenatide, Byetta, Bydureon, Tanzeum, Trulicity). To make certain Saxenda is safe for you, tell your health practitioner when you have:

• Stomach problems causing sluggish digestion;

• Kidney or liver disorder;

• High triglycerides (a form of fat in the blood);

• Heart troubles;

• a history of problems with your pancreas or gallbladder; or

• A history of depression or suicidal thoughts. In animal research, liraglutide caused thyroid tumors or thyroid most cancers. It isn't always acknowledged whether those consequences might occur in humans using ordinary doses. Ask your medical doctor approximately your risk. It isn't always known whether Saxenda will damage an unborn toddler. Tell your doctor in case you are pregnant or plan to become pregnant. It isn't recognised whether liraglutide passes into breast milk or if it could have an effect on the nursing infant. Tell your medical doctor if you are breast-feeding. Saxenda is not FDA-authorised for use through anyone younger than 18 years antique.

Before you begin Saxenda, your health practitioner will help you expand an extended-time period weight management plan. This need to include a low calorie diet and accelerated exercising. You can also paintings with a dietitian or nutritionist to increase your plan. Including Saxenda as a part of your plan can help you lose weight and keep it off long time. But unique human beings may additionally have distinctive outcomes with Saxenda. The amount of weight you can lose and any facet consequences you've got will depend upon your non-public situation. Saxenda's prescribing facts has information about facet outcomes and how much weight humans misplaced with Saxenda in research. But preserve in mind that everyone's enjoy with this drug could be special. To find out more approximately what you can assume with Saxenda, speak together with your medical doctor.